7 Days Green Smoothie Challenge for Weight Loss

Table of Contents

Disclaimer

This book has not been written by a doctor, healthcare professional or dietitian to offer medical advice.

You should check with your professional and private health advisor or doctor before starting your detox routine. The information of this book can't replace the guidance and attention of your physicians and healthcare professionals.

Every reader who wants to start 7-day green smoothie challenge should get the opinion of a qualified dietitian or health care professional or accept the whole responsibility if he/she decides to start without discussing it with his/her doctor.

The publishers and author of this book are not responsible for any decision that you will make after reading this smoothie challenge book.

Text Copyright © [Simone Higgins]

Legal & Disclaimer

The information contained in this book and its contents is not designed to replace or take the place of any form of medical or professional advice; and is not meant to replace the need for independent medical, financial, legal or other professional advice or services, as may be required. The content and information in this book has been provided for educational and entertainment purposes only.

The content and information contained in this book has been compiled from sources deemed reliable, and it is accurate to the best of the Author's knowledge, information and belief. However, the Author cannot guarantee its accuracy and validity and cannot be held liable for any errors and/or omissions. Further, changes are periodically made to this book as and when needed. Where appropriate and/or necessary, you must consult a professional (including but not limited to your doctor, attorney, financial advisor or such other professional advisor) before using any of the suggested remedies, techniques, or information in this book.

Upon using the contents and information contained in this book, you agree to hold harmless the Author from and against any damages, costs, and expenses, including any legal fees potentially resulting from the application of any of the information provided by this book. This disclaimer applies to any loss, damages or injury caused by the use and application, whether directly or indirectly, of any advice or information presented, whether for breach of contract, tort, negligence, personal injury, criminal intent, or under any other cause of action.

You agree to accept all risks of using the information presented inside this book.

You agree that by continuing to read this book, where appropriate and/or necessary, you shall consult a professional (including but not limited to your doctor, attorney, or financial advisor or such other advisor as needed) before using any of the suggested remedies, techniques, or information in this book.

BONUS: Free Gift Just for You

SIMONE HIGGINS

THE
MINDSET

THE MINDSET ALL
SUCCESSFUL PEOPLE
HAVE IN COMMON

Want to read another NEW e-book by Simone Higgins for FREE? Visit

http://simonehiggins.com/claim-your-free-gift/ to sign-up and receive another FREE copy of the best Simone Higgins books once it's available.

Introduction

Smoothies offer you more energy and make you happy and slim. If you are taking smoothies for the first time, it will take some time for your body to adjust to the new diet. Soon you will be habitual to eat green leaves because your body crave for it. Green leaves can boost the energy of your body with its nutrition.

Green leaves can make increase the alkaline level of your body. The modern diet is increasing acidification in your body. Eating a diet with alkaline is essential to make your body feel good. By including green salads and smoothies in your diet, you can give more rest to your digestive system. It allows your digestive system to use maximum energy for this whole procedure in your body. If you facilitate digestion, it will automatically leave maximum energy for other things.

Green smoothies are healthy to get rid of cellulite of your body, and it will be easy for you to get a flat stomach, shiny hair, and strong nails. You will get a fresh breath and get the healthy, tight and smooth skin. To get the healthy, lean and muscular body, introduce pure food in your life and open up the doorway to a spiritual life. A glass of green smoothie will help you to cleanse your body.

The scientific research shows that every cell in your body has its unique cosmos; therefore, it is healthy to fill yourself with pure food to let these cosmos flow through your body. If you want to see the miracles of pure food, make sure to avoid food that can increase the stress on your bodies, such as flour, white sugar, and caffeine. By reducing your weight with healthy food, you can sparkle your life with joy and happiness.

With the help of a plant-based healthy diet, you can reduce cholesterol level of your body. If you want to increase good cholesterol in your body, you should increase the consumption of green vegetables and citrus fruits in your diet. Unlike drinking fruit juices, the green smoothies consist of whole vegetables and fruit so that you can get nutrition and fiber. Fiber is essential for your colon health. It feeds your gut microbes, support optimum digestion and strong immune system. After adding green smoothies to your diet, you will notice a real change in your nails, skin, and hair. These will look healthy and strong. After drinking green smoothies, you will get glowing skin and clear up your adult acne.

Chapter 1 – Miracles of Green Smoothies for Natural Weight Loss

If you want to experience the unique benefits of green smoothies, you can follow the given steps:

- Increase the devour of green leaves that are high in the essential vitamins and minerals that are important for your body to function.
- You have to consume live enzymes that are proteins and act as a catalyst. Your body cells need live enzymes to repair them and build new healthy cells. Live enzymes can make your body shine.
- Green smoothies are good to increase the hydrochloric acid in the stomach that is important for the absorption and digestion of food.
- Green chlorophyll of leaves is encapsulated sunlight. Chlorophyll has a similar composition of human blood. The chlorophyll rich food is essential for the cleaning of your internal organs and blood. Cleaner blood will

decrease the burden on your organs that means you are at lower risk of getting diseases.

- The fiber in the green leaves can clear your bowels because undigested and old food in your bowel is a major villain behind your ill health. If your colon is functioning in a healthy way, you will get more energy.

Natural Weight Loss with Green Smoothies

Every person tries to get a slim body because they consider it ideal to live happily in the society. They run after some tricks, such as different crash diets, pills, and powders. These all methods will not work on your energy, strength of immunity system and happiness. Instead of running behind unhealthy ways to reduce weight, make sure to use natural items that can focus on your external and internal health. You can achieve it by changing your habits and lifestyles.

After achieving your ideal weight naturally, you will feel satisfying, powerful, strong, healthy, happy and energetic. You will feel your inside beauty. The green smoothies will help you to reach your ideal weight and maintain it in the future. Delicious green smoothies can satisfy your craving; hence, you will not feel hungry after having them in the morning or evening. After drinking smoothies, you can accomplish the feeling of satisfaction.

Increase Your Happiness

The intestine and the stomach are directly linked to your central nervous system and brain. Therefore, they reach quickly on your feelings and food choice. Some scientists consider stomach a second brain. Almost 95% of feel-good hormone serotonin is triggered by your stomach, and various gastrointestinal complaints are linked to stress. Green leaves are rich in fiber, and these are the basis for your green smoothies. These act as a sponge by removing and absorbing undigested toxins and foods that present in your gut.

Sauerkraut juice contains lots of beneficial bacteria that are essential for your stomach. To assist good bacteria in your stomach, you have to drink sauerkraut juice or eat a fermented vegetable on a regular basis. For quick and healthy weight loss, you have to get rid of animal products, dairy, flour, and sugar. These can make your bowl irritable and constipated by creating a buildup of undigested food. The green smoothies contain soluble fiber that can help you to clear your intestine. With a functioning gut, you will feel healthier and happy. When you lose some unwanted pounds, your body feels light and automatically become happy.

Chapter 2 – Healthy Green Smoothies to Cleanse Your Body

Detox and cleanse your body with delicious smoothies that are easy to prepare. You can add them in your regular routine. These smoothies can detox your body while providing important minerals, vitamins and all essential elements to your body. Here are some recipes of delicious and green smoothies. You will only need a blender and ingredients mentioned in the recipe. Blend all ingredients in blender or food processor and enjoy it:

Recipe 01: Green Protein Smoothie

Ingredients:

- Almond milk (unsweetened): ½ cup
- Almond butter: 1 tablespoon
- Banana: 1
- Mixed greens (spinach, chard and kale): 2 cups

Directions:

Put all ingredients in your food processor or blender and blend for almost 2 minutes to get a smooth mixture. Enjoy it in the breakfast.

Recipe 02: Glowing Green Smoothie

Ingredients:

- Kiwi: 1
- Banana: 1
- Chopped Pineapple: ¼ cup
- Celery stalks: 2
- Spinach: 2 cups
- Water: 1 cup

Directions:

Put all ingredients in your food processor or blender and blend for almost 2 minutes to get a smooth mixture. Enjoy it in the breakfast.

Recipe 03: Apple Berry Smoothie

Ingredients:

- Mixed berries (blueberries, strawberries and raspberries): 1 cup
- Large apple: 1
- Spinach: 2 cups
- Almond milk or water: 1 cup

Directions:

Put all ingredients in your food processor or blender and blend for almost 2 minutes to get a smooth mixture. Enjoy it.

Recipe 04: Pineapple Banana Smoothie

Ingredients:

- Pineapple: 1 cup
- Banana: 1
- Apple: 1
- Spinach: 2 cups
- Water: 1 cup

Directions:

Put all ingredients in your food processor or blender and blend for almost 2 minutes to get a smooth mixture. Enjoy it.

Detox with Kale

Kale is a superfood and packed with excellent amounts of minerals, vitamins and essential nutrients. Kale has a strong taste and you may not like it alone; therefore, it can be combined with other ingredients. Combination of kale with right ingredients will make it healthy and delicious. Make sure to use only leaves and discard its stems to avoid bitter flavor of kale.

Recipe 05: Apple and Kale Detox Smoothie

Ingredients:

- Unsweetened Almond milk: 2/3 cup
- Ice: ¾ cup
- Chopped kale: 1 ½ cups
- Chopped celery: 1 stalk
- Green or red apple (chopped and cored): ½
- Powdered Flax seed: 1 tablespoon
- Honey: 1 teaspoon

Directions:

Put all ingredients in your food processor or blender and blend for almost 2 minutes to get a smooth mixture. Enjoy it.

Recipe 06: Kale, Coconut and Pineapple Smoothie

Ingredients:

- Banana: 1
- Pineapple: 1 cup
- Coconut water: 1 cup
- Chopped kale: 2 cups

Directions:

Put all ingredients in your food processor or blender and blend for almost 2 minutes to get a smooth mixture. If you are not happy with the thickness, you can add some water to get desired consistency. Enjoy it.

Recipe 07: Strawberry and Kale Detox

Ingredients:

- Banana: 1
- Plain yogurt: 1 cup
- Fresh strawberries: 1 cup
- Chopped kale: 1 cup
- Ice: 1 cup

Directions:

Put all ingredients in your food processor or blender and blend for almost 2 minutes to get a smooth mixture. Enjoy it.

Recipe 08: Avocado Smoothie Recipe

Avocados ae super foods with lots of nutrients such as potassium, folate, and vitamins B, C and K. Consumption of avocado will help you to improve your cardiovascular health, promote eye health, relieve inflammation of joints, reduce weight and strengthen your bones.

Ingredients:

- Apple juice: 1 ½ cups
- Kale or spinach (chopped and stemmed): 2 cups
- Chopped and cored apple: 1
- Chopped Avocado: ½

Directions:

Put all ingredients in your food processor or blender and blend for almost 2 minutes to get a smooth mixture. Add water to get desired consistency. Enjoy it.

Recipe 09: Ultimate Detox Recipe

Ingredients:

- Peeled orange: 1
- Peeled banana: 1 medium
- Peeled lime: ½
- Chia seeds (soaked for five minutes): 1 tablespoon
- Grated ginger: 1 small piece
- Chopped dandelion greens or kale: 2 cups
- Almond milk or water: 8 ounces

Directions:

Add everything in blender except greens and hit pulse button for 2 to 3 minutes. Now add greens and blend it on high for almost 30 seconds to get a creamy texture of smoothie.

Recipe 10: Ginger Spice Smoothie

Ginger root can detox your body in a better way as compared to other ingredients. You can enjoy anti-inflammatory benefits of cinnamon in ginger smoothie.

Ingredients:

- Ginger root: 1 nub
- Cinnamon: 1 teaspoon
- Spinach: 1 handful
- Purified water: 1 cup

Directions:

Put all ingredients in your food processor or blender and blend for almost 2 minutes to get a smooth mixture. Make sure to mince ginger before adding it in the smoothie. Enjoy it.

Recipe 11: Cocoa Smoothie

Detox your body with cocoa and honey. The antioxidants of strawberries and cocoa will be really beneficial.

Ingredients:

- Cocoa powder: 1 tablespoon
- Coconut milk: ½ cup
- Strawberries: ½ cup
- Ice: 1 cup (for summer season)

Directions:

Put all ingredients in your food processor or blender and blend for almost 2 minutes to get a smooth mixture. Enjoy it.

Recipe 12: Cleansing Smoothie

Ingredients:

- Cucumber: ¼
- Handful spinach: ½
- Avocado: ½
- Celery stalk: 1
- Fresh mint: 2 sprigs
- Kiwifruit: 1
- Purified water: 1 cup
- Apple: ½
- Lemon: 1 squirt

Directions:

Put all ingredients in your food processor or blender and blend for almost 2 minutes to get a smooth mixture. Enjoy it.

Recipe 13: Orange Smoothie

Ingredients:

- Ripe banana: 1 small
- Frozen pineapple: ¾ cup
- Blood oranges (juiced): 2 (1/2 cup juice)
- Coconut milk: ¾ cup
- Lime juice: 2 to 3 tablespoon
- Frozen greens (spinach and kale): 2 handfuls

Directions:

Put all ingredients in your food processor or blender and blend for almost 2 minutes to get a smooth mixture. Enjoy it.

Recipe 14: Purple Smoothie

Ingredients:

- Apple Juice: 1 cup
- Frozen blueberries: 1 cup
- Peeled, sliced and cored Anjou pear: 1 cup
- Plain yogurt (low-fat): ½ cup
- Frozen strawberries: ½ cup
- Loosely packed kale (remove stems): ½ cup
- Flaxseed oil: 2 tablespoons
- Lemon juice: ½ lemon

Directions:

Put all ingredients in your food processor or blender and blend for almost 2 minutes to get a smooth mixture. Enjoy it.

Recipe 15: Special Detox Blend

Ingredients:

- Frozen banana: 1
- Ripe avocado: ½
- Kale (remove stem): 2 leaves
- Orange zest: ¼ teaspoon
- Matcha powder: 1 teaspoon
- Ginger powder: ½ teaspoon
- Kiwi fruit (remove skin): 1
- Coconut oil: 1 teaspoon
- Almond or coconut milk: ½ cup

Toppings:

- Pumpkin Seeds: 1 teaspoon
- Granola: 1 teaspoon
- Coconut shreds: 1 teaspoon
- Rose petals (dried): 1 teaspoon
- Blood orange: 3 slices to garnish

Directions:

Chop banana, kale and avocado and put them in the blender with remaining ingredients.

Now blend these ingredients to make a creamy and smooth mixture.

Pour this blend in a bowl and add desired toppings. Serve chilled.

Recipe 16: Beetroot Smoothie

Ingredients:

- Water: 1 cup
- Peeled and chopped beetroot: 1 small
- Cored and chopped apple: 1 small
- Peeled cucumber: ½
- Lemon juice: 1 tablespoon
- Shiro Miso: 1 tablespoon
- Chopped spring onion: 1 tablespoon
- Black pepper and Salt: as per taste
- Avocado pitted: ½ ripe

Toppings:

- Pumpkin seeds (you can take other seeds as well)
- Fresh dill
- Olive oil (extra-virgin) or Unsweetened Vegan Yogurt
- Black pepper: Freshly ground

Directions:

Combine cucumber, apple, beetroot, lemon juice, pepper, salt, spring onion, water and miso in a blender. Blend all ingredients to make them smooth.

Now add avocado and blend them once again. Taste and adjust the spices in this blend.

Serve chilled or normal after topping it with your favorite toppings.

Recipe 17: Mint and Watermelon Smoothie

Total Time: 15 minutes

Servings: 2

Ingredients:

- Chopped watermelon: 3 cups
- Strawberries: 1 cup
- Frozen cherries: ¾ cup
- Ginger root: 1 tablespoon
- Baobab powder: 1 teaspoon
- Cherry powder: 1 teaspoon
- Coconut milk: ¼ cup
- Mint leaves: 2 tablespoons
- Watermelon cubes: for garnishing

Directions:

Blend all ingredients in a blender to make a smooth mixture.

Pour in serving bowl or glasses and garnish with watermelon cubes, mint leaves and frozen fruit. Serve chilled.

Recipe 18: Coconut Curry Vegan Smoothie

Total Time: 15 minutes

Servings: 4

Ingredients:

- Thai coconut (young): 1 (1 cup flesh and 1.5 cups water)
- Chopped carrot: 1 thin
- Garlic: 1 clove
- Fresh Ginger: 1.5 teaspoon
- Curry powder: 2 teaspoon
- Chili pepper (Thai): ½ teaspoon (you can add more as per your taste)
- Chopped green onion: 2 tablespoons
- Julienned Persian cucumbers to make noodles: 2
- Red bell pepper: 1 (chop like matchsticks)
- Cilantro: 1 handful
- Water: ½ cup
- Lemon juice: ½ tablespoon
- Medjool date (pitted): 1

Directions:

Take one medium sized bowl and fill it with cilantro, cucumber noodles and bell pepper.

Blend remaining ingredients in your blender to make a smooth mixture. If you need warm soup, you can blend for 2 minutes; otherwise, blend to make a creamy mixture.

Pour this mixture over vegetables, garnish with cilantro and serve at room temperature

Chapter 3 – Salsa and Salad for Smoothie Challenge

If you want to enjoy salsa and salad with a unique twist, these recipes will prove really delicious for you:

Recipe 01: Fruit Salsa

Total Time: 20 minutes

Servings: 8

Ingredients:

- Peeled, diced and pitted avocado: 1
- Chopped and seeded habanero pepper: 1
- Fresh chopped cilantro: 1 tablespoon
- Juiced lime: 1
- Salt: as per taste
- Diced, peeled and seeded mango: 1 (optional)
- Chopped red onion: 1 small

Directions:

Put avocado in the serving bowl and mix them with lime juice. Mix in habanero pepper, onion and mango. Spice this salsa with salt and cilantro and serve chilled.

Recipe 02: Fruity Skewers

Total Time: 15 minutes

Servings: 5

Ingredients:

- Skewers: 20
- Peeled and chopped bananas: 2
- Chopped Cantaloupe: ¼
- Chopped apples: 1
- Halved strawberries: 5
- Grapes: 20 pieces

Directions:

Thread fruits on skewers in the following arrangement:

- Apple
- Banana
- Cantaloupe
- Strawberries
- Grapes

Put almost two pieces of fruits on every skewer. Arrange fruit skewers on your serving plates and serve.

Recipe 03: Walnut, Avocado and Cranberry Salad

Total Time: 30 minutes

Servings: 4

Ingredients:

- Baby spinach: 3 cups
- Sliced, cored and peeled green apples: 2 medium
- Sliced avocado: 1 medium
- Walnuts: 1 cup
- Dried cranberries: 1/3 cup

Dressing:

- Coconut Balsamic vinegar: ¼ cup
- Honey: 2 teaspoons
- Dijon mustard: ½ teaspoon
- Black pepper and sea salt: 1 pinch

Directions:

Mix dressing ingredients in one bowl and whisk them well to combine.

Take another bowl and add salad ingredients to this bowl. Pour dressing over salad ingredients before serving it.

Recipe 04: Salad with Lime Dressing

Total Time: 15 minutes

Servings: 4

Ingredients:

Salad:

- Mixed greens: 11 ounces
- Diced mango: 1
- Diced and peeled avocado: 1
- Sliced bell pepper: 1 red
- Sliced bell pepper: 1 orange
- Minced parsley: ¼ cup
- Sprouted or raw pepitas: 1/3 cup
- Honey and lime dressing: as per taste

Dressing:

- Olive oil: ¾ cup
- Lime juice: 4 ½ tablespoons
- Honey: 1 ½ tablespoons
- Dijon mustard: 1 ½ teaspoons
- Red pepper crushed flakes: ½ teaspoon

- Minced garlic: 1 clove

- Pepper and sea salt: as per taste

Directions:

Mix dressing ingredients in one bowl and whisk them well to combine.

Take another bowl and add salad ingredients to this bowl. Pour dressing over salad ingredients before serving it.

Recipe 05: Kale Salad

Total Time: 15 minutes

Servings: 4

Ingredients:

- Rice vinegar: ¼ cup
- Black pepper: ground as per taste
- Salt: as per taste
- Kale: 1 bunch
- Orange juice: 1 tablespoon
- Sliced persimmon: 1
- Dijon mustard: 1 teaspoon
- Apple cut like Matchsticks: 1
- Chopped and peeled orange: 2
- Ground cumin: 1 teaspoon
- Grated zest of orange: 1 teaspoon
- Pistachio nuts (chopped): ¼ cup
- Red pepper (flakes): ¼ teaspoon
- Olive oil: 1/3 cup

Directions:

Take one bowl and whisk pepper flakes, cumin, orange zest, Dijon mustard, orange juice and vinegar in this bowl. Slowly mix olive oil in the orange juice blend and whisk until combined. Season this mixture with black pepper and salt.

Remove stems of every kale leaf and stack 3 – 4 kale leaves. Roll them together and make fine crosswise slices of kale leaves to create ribbons.

Now combine pistachio nuts, orange, apple, persimmon, and sliced kale in one bowl. Add dressing and toss them well to coat everything. Serve chilled.

Recipe 06: Raw Salad

Total Time: 30 minutes

Servings: 4

Ingredients:

- Zucchini (trim ends): 2
- Carrots: 2
- Finely Chopped red cabbage: 1 head
- Finely chopped Red bell pepper: 1
- Bean sprouts: 1/2 cup
- Almond butter (raw): 3/4 cup
- Juiced oranges: 2
- Raw honey: 2 tablespoons
- Minced ginger root: 1 tablespoon
- Raw soy sauce or Nama Shoyu: 1 tablespoon
- Unpasteurized miso: 1 tablespoon
- Minced garlic: 1 clove
- Cayenne pepper: 1/4 teaspoon

Directions:

Make lengthwise slices of zucchini with the help of vegetable peeler to make thin and long noodles. Put these noodles on serving plates.

Make long strips of carrot with vegetable peeler to make long noodles similar to zucchini.

Combine beans sprouts, bell pepper, cabbage and carrots in one large bowl.

Take a separate bowl and whisk cayenne pepper, garlic, miso, nama shoyu, ginger, honey, orange juice and almond butter in this bowl. Keep this sauce aside.

Pour nearly half sauce in the cabbage mixture and toss well to coat. Top zucchini with cabbage blend and pour remaining sauce on every portion.

Recipe 07: Kelp Noodles with Ginger Pesto

Total Time: 30 minutes

Servings: 6

Ingredients:

Pesto

- Loosely packed mint leaves: ¾ cup
- Avocado oil: 3 tablespoons
- Chopped or minced ginger: 1 teaspoon
- Raw almonds: ¼ cup
- Garlic cloves: 3 to 4
- Chopped jalapeno: 1 teaspoon
- Raw honey: 1 teaspoon
- Sea salt: ½ teaspoon

Noodle Salad

- Chopped carrots: ½ cup
- Corn Kernels (raw): ½ cup
- Sea salt: 1 pinch
- Avocado oil: 1 teaspoon
- Juiced lemon: 1

- Kelp noodles: 12 ounces
- Baking soda: 1 teaspoon

Directions:

Make Pesto:

Process all ingredients of pesto in your food ingredients by pulsing it for almost 1 minute. Scrape all the sides of bowl and keep this pesto aside.

Veggie and Noodles

Take one bowl of medium size and mix kelp noodles with baking soda and half of the lemon juice. It will make noodles soft.

Mix noodles with your hands and coat well in baking soda and lemon juice. Keep them aside while prepare remaining dish. Keep mixing them by your hands with frequent intervals to make them soft. Before mixing them with rest of the ingredients, make sure to rinse them properly.

Take one bowl and add avocado oil, corn, carrots, lemon juice and sea salt in this bowl. Toss it to coat all ingredients. Add noodles to this mixture (make sure to rinse noodles and dry them before adding in the bowl).

Top with some mint pesto and garnish with almonds and mint. Serve normal or chilled.

Recipe 08: Cauliflower Rice

Total Time: 30 minutes

Servings: 4

Ingredients:

- Chopped and washed cauliflower: 1 head
- Olive oil: 1 tablespoon
- Chili powder: ½ teaspoon
- Cumin: 1 to 2 teaspoons (based on the size of cauliflower head)
- Pink Salt: ½ teaspoon
- Diced tomato: 1 large
- Diced red onion: ¾
- Chopped cilantro: 1 handful
- Lime juice: ½ lime juiced
- Chopped green onion: 3 sprigs

Directions:

Put chili powder, salt, cumin, and cauliflower in a food processor. Pulse these ingredients until you get the consistency of rice.

Put the cauliflower rice in one bowl with remaining ingredients and carefully fold all ingredients to combine everything well.

Serve with your favorite sauce.

Chapter 4 – 7 Days Green Smoothie Challenge for Weight Loss

If you want to reduce your weight within seven days, you can try it without starving because fresh fruits and vegetables are available. You can start with this sample plan:

Day 01:

>**Breakfast:** 32-ounce carrot juice

>**Lunch:** 16-ounce smoothie to flush fat

>**Dinner:** 16-ounce smoothie to flush fat

Day 02:

>**Breakfast:** 32-ounce carrot juice

>**Lunch:** 16-ounce smoothie to flush fat

>**Dinner:** 16-ounce smoothie to flush fat

Day 03:

>**Breakfast:** 32-ounce Detox Juice

>**Lunch:** 16-ounce smoothie to flush fat

Dinner: Vegetable salad (unlimited)

Day 04:

Breakfast: 32-ounce Carrot Juice

Lunch: 16-ounce smoothie to flush fat

Dinner: Vegetable salad (unlimited)

Day 05:

Breakfast: 32-ounce Detox Juice

Lunch: 16-ounce smoothie to flush fat

Dinner: 16-ounce smoothie to flush fat

Day 06:

Breakfast: 32-ounce Carrot Juice

Lunch: 16-ounce smoothie to flush fat

Dinner: Vegetable salad (unlimited)

Day 07:

Breakfast: 32-ounce Carrot Juice

Lunch: 16-ounce smoothie to flush fat

Dinner: Vegetable salad (unlimited)

Recipes Mentioned in the Diet Plan

Recipe 01: Carrot Juice

Ingredients:

- Granny Smith medium apples: 2
- Ginger: 1 to 2 knuckles
- Carrots: 3 cored and chopped

Directions:

Blend all ingredients in your blender and enjoy this healthy breakfast.

Recipe 02: Detox Juice

Ingredients:

- Cilantro or parsley: 1 bunch
- Ginger: 1 knuckle
- Whole lemon: 1
- Kale or spinach: 2 to 3 handfuls
- Granny smith medium apples: 2
- Cucumbers or celery: 2 or more to make 32-ounce juice

Directions:

Blend all ingredients in your blender to get a consistent and smooth mixture.

Recipe 03: Smoothie to Flush Fat (16-ounce)

Ingredients:

- Granny smith medium apple: 1 (Cored)
- Romaine lettuce: 2 mounding cups
- Kale or spinach: 1 to 2 handfuls
- Cucumber: ½ or celery: 2 to 3 sticks
- Lemon juice: ½ lemon (squeeze to get fresh juice)
- Coconut water: as per need
- Organic stevia (as per need): optional

Directions:

Blend all ingredients in your blender to get a consistent and smooth mixture. If you want to make 32-ounce smoothie, make sure to double the ingredients.

Recipe 04: Salad

To make salad, you can choose non-starchy vegetables and leafy greens. There is no need to add corn in the salad.

Ingredients:

- Chopped bell pepper: 1 cup
- Chopped tomatoes: 1 cup
- Chopped broccoli: 1 cup
- Chopped Onion: ½ cup
- Chopped carrot: 1 cup
- Chopped celery: 1 cup
- Chopped cucumber: 1 cup
- Chopped cauliflower: 1 cup

Directions:

Mix all ingredients in a bowl and mix in salad dressing to enhance its taste.

Recipe 05: Avocado Dressing

Ingredients:

- Avocado: ½
- Zucchini: ½
- Cilantro: 1 handful
- Garlic: 1 clove
- Apple cider vinegar: as per taste
- Water: as per need to get required texture

Directions:

Blend all ingredients in your bowl and mix it with your vegetable salad.

Recipe 06: Low Fat Pepper Dressing

Ingredients:

- Zucchini: ½
- Red bell pepper: ½
- Parsley or cilantro: 1 handful
- Garlic: 1 clove
- Lemon juice: squeeze 1 lemon
- Jalapeno: 1 teaspoon (optional)

Directions:

Blend all ingredients in a bowl to get consistent and smooth mixture. Pour it over salad and enjoy.

Chapter 5 – Tips to Continue Losing Weight and Maintain Good Health Afterwards

After losing weight, it is time for celebration because weight loss is not easy, but keeping all those pounds off will be a real challenge for you. If you want to continue losing weight and maintain good health after your smoothie challenge, you should say good bye to your bad habits. Make sure to change your habits on permanent basis. Here are some ways for your assistance.

Discover Actual Reason of Overeating

Just look back at your bad habits and find out the reasons of overeating in your past. It is essential to understand either you are habitual to eat food to decrease your stress. Some overeating triggers may have links with hormones. Some PMS hormonal changes can make you crave for salty or sweet food. Your mood can be another factor to trigger your hunger. If you are depressed, you may like to eat food to get rid of depression.

Plan for Your Success

You should make a regular budget for daily meals, such as snacks. Your regular meals plate should contain one quarter legumes or meat as a protein source, one quarter starch, such as pasta or rice and 2 servings of colored vegetables on almost half of your plate. Type of food can influence your hunger feelings. Avoid overeating of carbohydrates and increase protein content in your diet.

Keep An Eye on Portions

The portion size is really important because large portion size can increase your weight. There is no need to enjoy five portions of ice cream because you will gain weight. Control your craving and control your portion size, even while eating healthy food. Use a small plate and fill it with food to satisfy your hunger.

Keep Using Your Scale

After reducing weight, people often keep their weighing scale aside. It is not a good habit because you will always need your scale. Check your weight once a week to keep an eye on the transition of weight. If you have gained 1 to 2 pounds, focus on your portions. It is hard to find out if you are retaining water or actually gaining weight. If you are retaining fluid, you will feel your shoes and ring tight. The tight waistband of your jeans can be a reason of fluid retention or excessive food. Make sure to regularly step on the scale to keep an eye on your weight to avoid any weight gain.

Exercise for Almost 30 Minutes

After losing weight, you will still need a good session of sweat to manage your weight. To keep your extra pounds off, you should do regular exercise and avoid regaining these pounds. You should do exercise for almost 30 minutes in a day. You can increase the duration and intensity of your workout to challenge your body.

80/20 Rule is Good for Everyone

Losing your weight and keeping it off for a longer period of time is not a piece of cake. You have to do additional efforts. It will be good to follow 80/20 rule. This rule requires you to practice healthy habits for 80% of your time and relax for 20% of time. Keep it in mind that unhealthy meals can undo all your hard work. Keep an eye on your calories, eat healthy and live an active life to stay always slim. Drink plenty of water and stay always positive to improve your health.

Conclusion

One of the best ways to lose weight is the use of natural and healthy food items and exercise. You have to control your portion size and go for a walk on a regular basis. You have to need to follow Ketogenic diet. A simple rule of thumb is to eat real food, such as meat, nuts, eggs, yogurt, fruits and vegetables. There are a few things that you should eat during Ketogenic diet:

You may often hear that water can help you to shed few pounds, and it is true because of the miraculous properties of water. If you eat fruits and vegetables with water, then you can reduce the body mass and waistline. The water will fill you up to make you eat less amount of food. You have to include at least 90% water in your diet, and it is easy by consuming season fruits and vegetables with water.

Broccoli is an excellent source of fiber and calcium; therefore, you can add it to your salad and soups to shed some extra pounds. The cabbage has antioxidant properties with lots of vitamin C. It can boost your metabolism and trigger weight loss speed. You can pair raw cabbage with apple, orange juice, and chicken to make a yummy and healthy salad.

Like any other cruciferous vegetable, the cauliflower is good for cancer patients. It has vitamin C, folate, and phytonutrients, and it should be included in your regular diet. If you want to get rid of fat, you can consume raw cauliflower or roast it to increase its antioxidant power.

Leaf vegetables are excellent foods to consume because of low calories and fiber content. These are rich in iron, calcium, folate, vitamin K and lutein. These will help you to improve your bowel movements and reduce the risk of various diseases. You can consume cabbage, sprouts, cucumbers and broccoli on a regular basis.

You need calcium to prevent fat cells in the body, and the yogurt will help you a lot. It can reduce cholesterol, obesity, and high blood pressure. The yogurt can facilitate your weight loss process by enhancing your metabolism and support your immune system. The yogurt can supply plenty of proteins and vitamins in your body. If you want to get rid of extra kilos, you have to incorporate these food items in your diet. Go for a morning walk on a regular basis to burn more calories than you consume.

BONUS REMAINDER

SIMONE HIGGINS

THE
MINDSET

THE MINDSET ALL
SUCCESSFUL PEOPLE
HAVE IN COMMON

THE END

Enjoy what you read? Please leave a review on
Amazon. Thanks!

Want to read another NEW e-book by Simone

Higgins for FREE? Visit

http://simonehiggins.com/claim-your-free-gift/ to

sign-up and receive another FREE copy of the best

Simone Higgins books once its available.

Printed in Great Britain
by Amazon